Making Organic
Cosmetics

from your
Kitchen

100% Organic Beauty Recipes for healthier
Hair, Face and Body

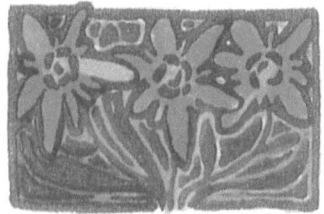

Andrea Hersey

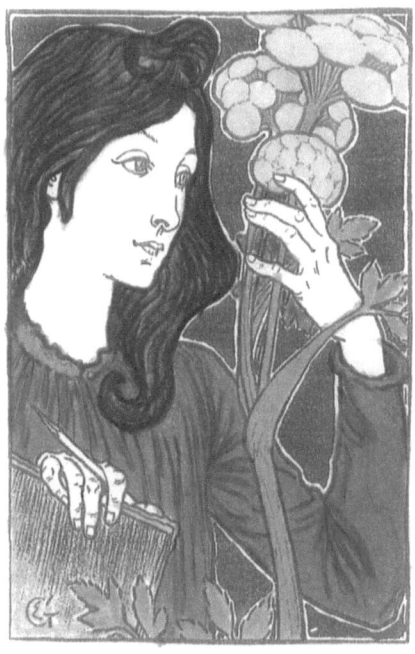

To order additional copies of this book, contact:
Xlibris Corporation
1-888-795-4274
www.Xlibris.com
Orders@Xlibris.com
73505

CONTENTS

Preface

One of the greatest treasures in life is HEALTH. In a healthy state, we are able to develop our lives in whichever direction we choose. Health is achieved by the effort to take care of ourselves acknowledging our reality in our immediate environment. Our daily activities, habits, relationships, work, and our own perception of all of the above potentially affect our health. We should evaluate what we feed to our senses, body, soul, and mind.

We need to be aware that we have been feeding our skin chemicals, alcohols, paints, and all sorts of preservatives, that only serve the purpose of a longer shelf life awaiting consumption. It is important to be aware that the cost of mass produced cosmetics includes bottling, labeling, electric, freight, laborers, oil, and many other expenses that the industry has, that you ignore and don't care to know about. Making our own cosmetics at home empowers our independence and creativity, provides us knowledge, connects us to nature, and brings us the opportunity to conserve and recycle.

For all your recipes you'll need to recycle your old bottles, make-up containers, cream containers and old cosmetics recipients. Your energy expense will include seconds to 1 minute in the microwave and 15 to 60 minutes on stove preparations. All these benefits, plus the discovery your senses will awake to, as you experiment with essential oils with rich aromatic fragrances that will indulge you as you use your own handmade preparations. This experience is beyond enjoyable! The costs of ingredients will not be so high and it will be more pleasant for you when you find out how little of each ingredient you use for each preparation.

This book is inspired in the urge for human beings to re-connect with nature and themselves. It seeks to lead women to enjoy the healthy benefits of making their own shampoos, conditioners, lip balms and lipsticks, face and body moisturizers, and other beneficial cosmetics from the comfort of their kitchens, perhaps the beauty of their gardens or the natural state of the ingredients. It also seeks to make women aware of the power and perfection of nature. I warranty that once you follow this recipes, you will never want to buy a mass produced cosmetic again. You will find that it is not only cheaper, but very beneficial for your skin, hair, mind, body and soul and you will glow with radiance and beauty.

Women!!! Do not put more carcinogens in your skin!!! Don't trade your health for anything! Awareness is the key to evolution; never think you are running out of time. Take the time to understand what you are consuming and how does this affect your body, mind, soul, and overall health.

General Electric's Advice:

Microwaved water and other liquids do not always bubble when they reach the boiling point. They can actually get superheated and not bubble at all. The superheated liquid will bubble up out of the cup when it is moved or when something like a spoon or tea bag is put into it.

To prevent this from happening and causing injury, **do not heat any liquid for more than two minutes per cup. After heating, let the cup stand in the microwave for thirty seconds! before moving it or adding anything into it.**

Here is what our local science teacher had to say on the matter: 'Thanks for the microwave warning. I have seen this happen before. It is caused by a phenomenon known as super heating. It can occur anytime water is heated and will particularly occur if the vessel that the water is heated in is new, or when heating a small amount of water (less than half a cup).

What happens is that the water heats faster than the vapor bubbles can form. If the cup is very new then it is unlikely to have small surface scratches inside it that provide a place for the bubbles to form. As the bubbles cannot form and release some of the heat has built up, the liquid does not boil, and the liquid continues to heat up well past its boiling point.

What then usually happens is that the liquid is bumped or jarred, which is just enough of a shock to cause the bubbles to rapidly form and expel the hot liquid. The rapid formation of bubbles is also why a carbonated beverage spews when opened after having been shaken.'

Hair

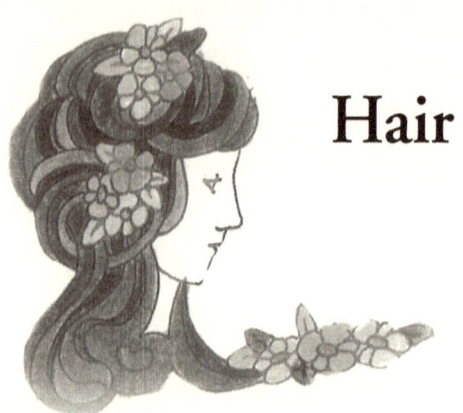

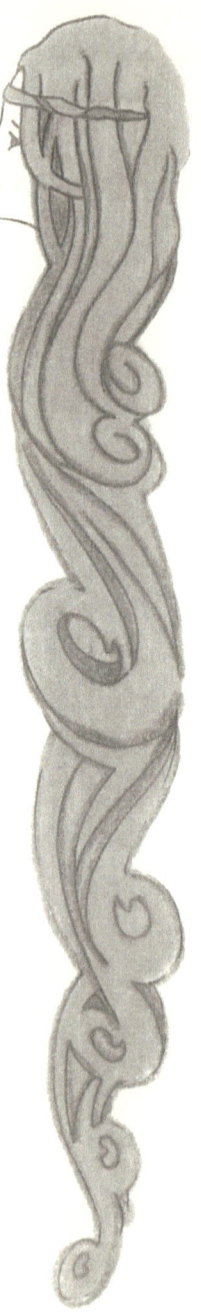

All Natural Shampoo

Blend the following Ingredients:

1 oz. Olive oil
1 egg
1 Tbsp. lemon juice
1 tsp. apple cider vinegar

Chamomile Shampoo

Make an Herbal Infusion with

4 cups of boiling water
5 Tbsp. of chamomile flower or Chamomile tea bags

Cover and Steep for 30 minutes. Strain and add:

4oz. Castile soap flakes or 2 oz. Castile soap or add baby shampoo.

Rosemary Hair Wash

¼ cup of dried Rosemary
1 ½ cups of water
1 tsp Baking Soda

Bring the water to a boil. Simmer Rosemary amount.
Add the Baking soda.
You can replace rosemary by chamomile, or sage.

Mild Shampoo

½ oz. soapwort root (crushed and dried)
½ oz. chamomile dried flower or 1 tea bag of chamomile
2 pints of water

-Bring water to a boil.
-Put the soapwort and the chamomile flowers into a bowl.
-Pour boiling water over the herbs.
-Steep for 15 minutes.
-Cool and Strain.

This amount will be sufficient for approximately 4 washes. Keep left over in the refrigerator.

Herbal Shampoo

A few bay leaves
A Handful of dried chamomile flowers or 2 bags of chamomile tea
A Handful of Rosemary leaves
1 Lt or 1 ¾ pints of boiling water
1 tsp of liquid soap (Baby shampoo)

Steep herbs in boiling water and add liquid soap amount. Apply. Rinse with water.

Egg Shampoo

2 small eggs
2 oz. of water
1 Tbsp. Apple cider vinegar or lemon juice.
Optional: 5 drops of Rosemary, or Rose, or Lavender essential oil, or any aroma that you enjoy. All this 3 essential oils are very aromatic as well as moisturizing for the hair.

Mix. Blend for 30 seconds at low speed. Massage into the scalp and rinse very thoroughly using lukewarm water.

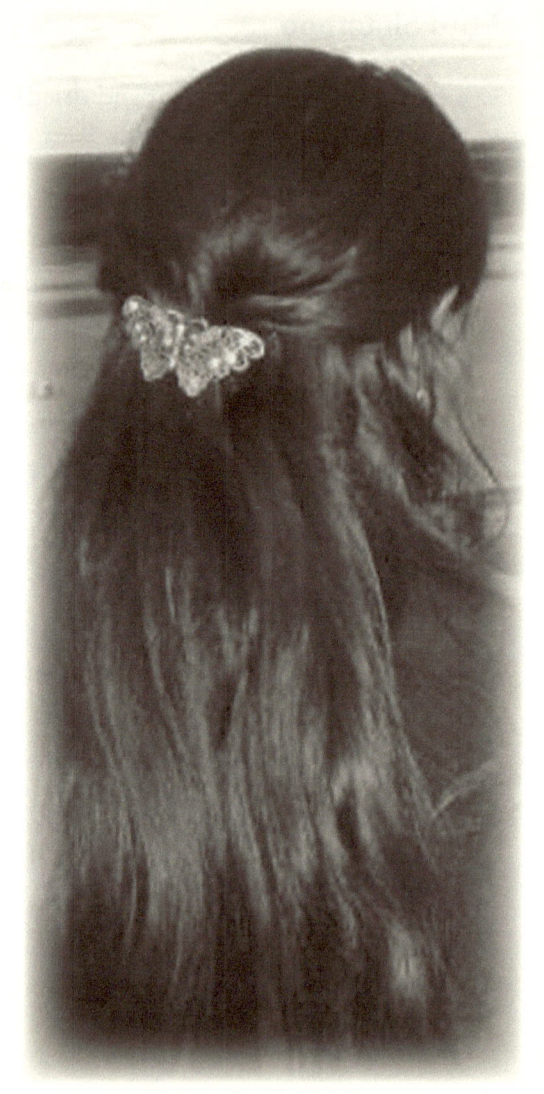

Soapwort and
Lemon shampoo

1 cup of soapwort or ritha nuts
1 tbsp fresh lemon juice

-Soak the ritha nuts or the soapwort nuts in a cup of water overnight.
-The next day, strain the liquid and mix in the lemon juice.
-Apply to the hair in the usual way and rinse with water.

Ritha; available in Indian shops. Soapwort cleans the hair thoroughly without producing lather. The lemon juice helps control oil secretion in a greasy scalp.

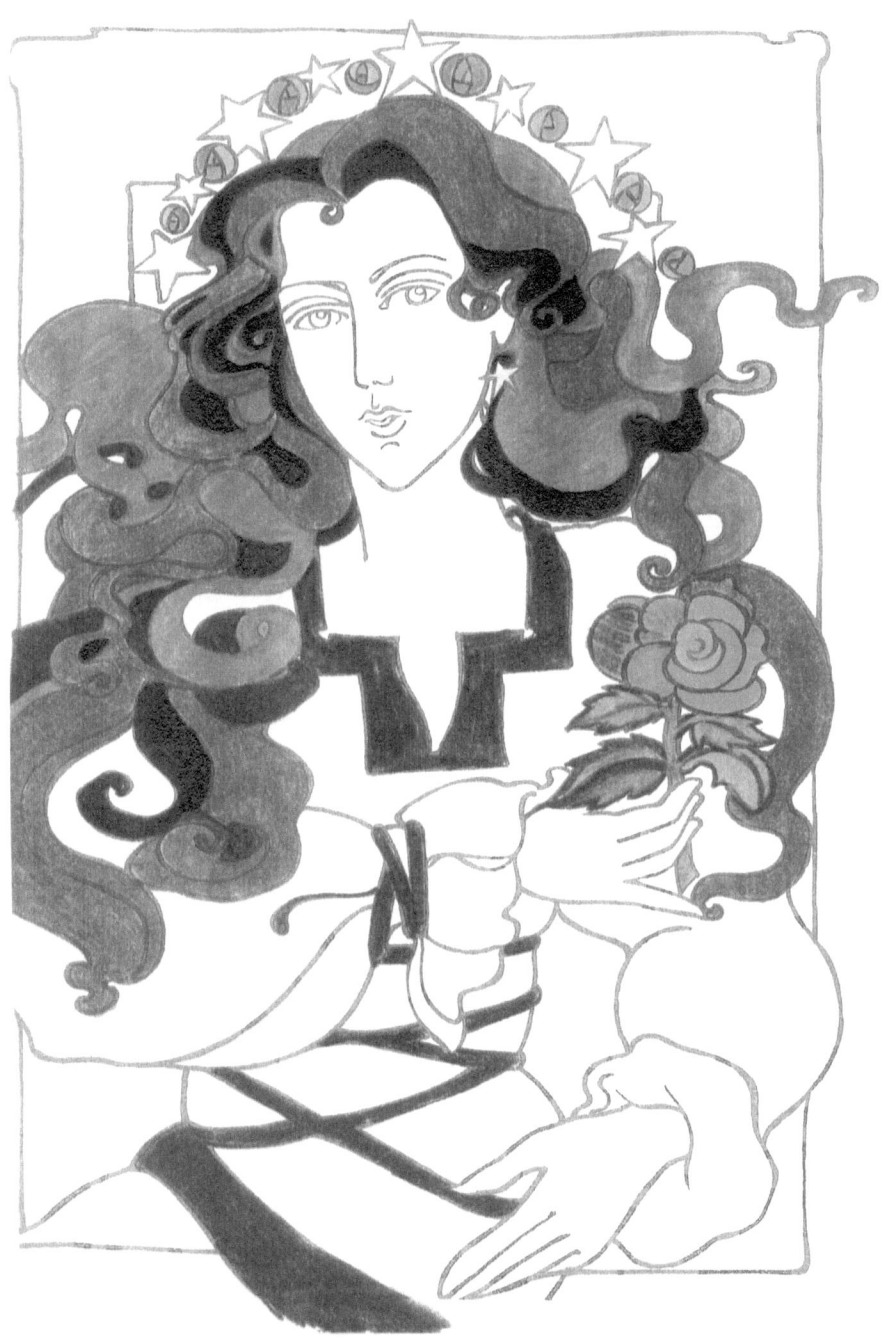

Ingredient Talk

Apple Cider Vinegar

Helps cleanse the hair, removing residue and buildup left over from every day shampoos, conditioners and hair products. It also helps to balance the PH of the Scalp and Hair. It also contains malic acid, which aids in the removal of dead skin cells. It is a traditional hair rinse when diluted in water.

Eggs

It is a source of high quality protein and a good source of 11 essential nutrients. Amongst them, Vitamin A & D, Choline, Carotenoids, Lutein, and Zeaxanthin.

Lemon

It was used by the Ancient Egyptians to clean their hair and scalps. Its acid cuts the oil and seals the cuticle to leave hair shiny and smelling fresh. It's a high source of Vitamin C, the best of anti-oxidants. It has bleaching properties, it can be used on the hair to enhance blonde highlights. It is highly antiseptic and has an astringent effect on the skin. It may be used to treat boils, broken capillaries, greasy skin, herpes and insect bites.

Baking Soda

Reduces hair oil and cleans up product build up.

Rosemary

(Rosmarinus Officinalis) It's volatile oils have strong antiseptic properties. It makes an excellent rinse for the hair. Rosemary essential oil is refreshing and stimulating. It is excellent for hair and scalp problems, including hair loss and dandruff.

Sage

(Salvia officinalis) Is an antiseptic to the skin and darkens the hair. It is also useful in the treatment of Dandruff. Sage relieves excessive sweating. Sage essential oil has a fresh, herbaceous and camphoraceous smell. It is strongly stimulating.

Chamomile

Chamomile flowers help to keep blonde hair a bright clear color. They will not lift the color that is medium to dark, but will help brighten naturally fair hair as well as leaving a pleasant fragrance. The healing properties of chamomile are antifungal, antibacterial, anti-inflammatory and anti-allergenic.

Olive oil

Olive oil consists of triglycerides or oleic, linoleic and palmitic acids, and it is used as an emollient and as a soap base. It is soothing, nourishing and lubricant.

Soapwort root

(Saponaria officinalis) Infusions of soapwort have been used as a cleanser for the hair and skin for centuries. In India, it is called "ritha." When boiled in water it gives a froathy, soapy infusion.

Hair Conditioners

Basic Hair Conditioner

¼ cup oil of either: Olive Oil
Jojoba Oil
Sweet Almond Oil
Castor Oil

10 drops total of essential oils of Lavender, Rosemary and Basil or either of these by itself.
Work the mixture in your hair, leave in for 10 minutes, and rinse with shampoo.

Avocado and Mayo Conditioner

1 cup of mayonnaise
1 ripe avocado or replace by ½ cup of avocado oil

-Mash avocado very well with a fork and add the mayonnaise (you may want to use the blender to give it a more creamy texture).
-Work the mixture into your hair, covering your head with a plastic cap.
-Let the mixture sit for 15-20 minutes and rinse thoroughly with water.

Mashed Banana conditioner

Mash 1 ripe banana, the riper the better.
Work it into your hair.
Rinse thoroughly with water

Dark Hair conditioner

Amla oil or dried gooseberry oil

-After shampooing your hair, pour 2 drops of Amla oil into your hands.
-Rub hands together, greasing them lightly.
-Rub your hands into your hair, try to work your hair as if you were combing it with your hands and detangling it.
-Rinse your hair . . . . wherever you feel your hair is tangly, grease your hands again with a little bit of Amla oil and apply on to that section.

Light Hair Conditioner

-Jasmin oil
-After shampooing your hair, pour 4 drops of Jasmin oil into your hands.
-Rub hands together, greasing them.
-Rub your hands into your hair, try to work your hair as if you were combing it with your hands and detangling it.
-Rinse your hair . . . . wherever you feel your hair is tangly, grease your hands again with a little bit of Jasmin oil and apply on to that section.

Herb infused oils

Herb of your choice, chamomile for light hair, rosemary, lavender or sage for dark hair for example.
2 cups of olive oil, coconut or jojoba oil, either one
Double boiler

Place your carrier oil in the top pot of your double boiler and mix in the herbs. Let the heat of the boiling below, steep the herbs into the oil. Once the oil is perfumed with the herbs, take out and strain. Bottle the oil and use it as a conditioner, in the same manner as the Jasmin or Amla oil conditioners.

Leave-in Conditioner

4 oz. of water
8 drops of any essential oil that suits your hair and need.

You can use: Rosemary if you have dark hair, Rose, or geranium rose, to moisturize, Lavender to detangle and for the aroma, Sage or Tea Tree oil to combat dandruff and darken your hair. Or any others you prefer . . . You can also use Amla or Jasmin Hair oil, pouring only some drops into the amount given of water given above. Put this mixture into a spray bottle or a spritzer.

Hair Treatments

Stimulating Hair Oil

-Double Boiler Pot
-4 oz. Avocado oil
-1/4 cup Basil Leaves
-1/4 cup of Rosemary leaves

-Prepare the bottom of the double boiler with the water you are to boil. In the top pot pour the Avocado oil along with the Basil and Rosemary leaves.
Note: These ones could be fresh or dried. If you are going to gather them from your garden, make sure you pick the leaves from the tips of your plants.
-Put a lid to the top mixture and let the oil heat up. The herbs will saturate the oil with their aroma.
-Leave for 30 minutes until you notice the oil smells like basil and rosemary.
-Let the mixture cool, strain, and bottle.
-Massage the mixture into your scalp.
-Leave-in for 30 minutes, you may want to wear a plastic cap for better absorption. Then wash your hair with mild shampoo.

Hair mask for extra Conditioning

½ of a ripe banana
¼ avocado or replace by 1 Tbsp of Avocado oil
1 Tbsp of wheat germ oil
1 Tbsp natural plain yogurt
¼ tsp of vitamin E oil.

Mix all the ingredients above. Apply mixture in the hair and leave in for 15 minutes. Rinse thoroughly and Shampoo.

Anti-Frizz Pomade

2 Tbsp Amla oil or dried gooseberry oil
1 Tbsp Castor oil
1 Tbsp Beeswax

-Chip the beeswax to the amount listed above and place inside a glass container (0.25 oz. or 0.38 oz) This recipient could be recycled from and old tub of lip gloss, or a small cream container that is already empty.
-Mix the Amla and Castor oil. Put the container with the mixture inside the microwave and heat for about 20 seconds or until you see that the beeswax has melted completely.
-Take out making sure you don't burn your fingers, cap, and put in the freezer to harden.
-Wait 30 minutes to an hour, and your pomade will be made.

Dab a little bit, rub your fingers and apply on to the frizzy hair, Do not put to much . . . .

Fragrant Hair Sheen

12 oz of purified water
5 drops of rosemary essential oil
5 drops of Lavender essential oil

-Mix all ingredients above.
-After the shampoo shake and pour mixture in your hair. Make sure you don't waste a bit, neither pour too much.
-Feel your hair, if it feels oily, rinse with abundant water. If your hair feels smooth and good to comb, don't rinse too much with water rather leave in.

Ingredient Talk

Avocado

(Persea Americana) The fruit of the tree is naturally rich in unsaturated oils which hydrate, nourish and moisturize the skin. Avocado oil is an excellent emollient and natural colorant. It contains oleic, linoleic and palmitic acids.

Banana

(Musa acuminata) The fruit contains high levels of vitamins and minerals, especially Potassium. It is humectant and moisturizing.

Wheatgerm oil

This heavy rich oil is a natural source of vitamin E. It is a heavy oil in the real sense of the word and thus often is combined with a lighter oil such as Almond oil. It also has a distinctive odor. It is very effective in the treatment of wrinkles and stretch marks.

Yogurt

Produced by the action of bacteria in milk, yogurt cleanses and conditions the skin and is readily absorbed. It contains lactic acid which is thought to stimulate cell production.

Vitamin E

Antioxidants such as vitamin E act to protect our cells against the effects of free radicals, which are potentially damaging by-products of energy metabolism. Free radicals can damage cells and may contribute to the development of cardiovascular disease and cancer.

Amla Hair Oil or dried gooseberry oil

Amla (**Emblica officinalis**) is an extensively used herb in making ayurvedic medicines. It keeps us away from all the diseases by boosting our immune system. It is the richest natural source of vitamin C. It stimulates hair follicles thus promoting hair growth and also improves hair texture. It prevents premature graying of hairs and dandruff. **Amla** acts as natural hair conditioner and provides good nourishment. Dabur Amla Hair Oil combines the goodness of amla fruit (Indian gooseberry) with a blend of vegetable and mineral oils to promote long, healthy hair. Regular application can assist in reducing split ends and minor hair loss. Dabur Amla Hair Oil has been the secret of beautiful hair in India and around the world for over 50 years.

-Massage your scalp with Dabur Amla hair oil leave overnight for best results shampoo next morning to get healthy and lustrous hair.

Jasmin Hair oil

For ages, the enchanting fragrance of Jasmine has spellbound people. Dabur Jasmine Hair Oil has the same fragrant goodness of Jasmine. It gives your hair new life and makes it long, thick and beautiful.

Castor Oil

This thick, colorless oil provides a protective, waterproof coating to both the skin and hair.

Beeswax

Wax produced by the Honey Bee (Apis Mellifera), which contains a mixture of fatty acids and esters. It is used in a range of cosmetics and toiletries as a thickener and emulsifier.

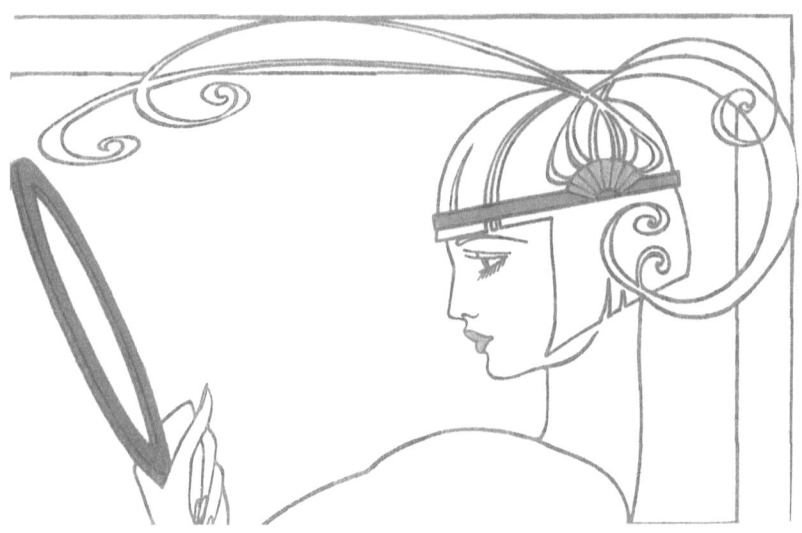

Eyes, Eyebrows and Eyelashes

Treatment

2 Tbsp Amla oil
1 Tbsp Castor oil
1 Tbsp Beeswax
1 glass container (0.25 oz. or 0.38 oz). This recipient could be recycled from and old tub of lip gloss, or a small cream container that is already empty.

-Chip the beeswax to the amount listed above and pour the Amla and Castor oil in the container.
-Place the mixture in the microwave and heat for about 20 seconds or until you see that the beeswax has melted completely.
-Take out making sure you don't burn your fingers, cap, and put in the freezer to harden.
-Wait 30 minutes to an hour, and your pomade will be made.

Apply this mixture to your eyebrows and eyelashes at night before going to sleep.

Healing oil mixture for Eyebrows

½ tsp vegetable oil
½ tsp castor oil
2-3 drops of camphor oil
.025 oz plastic or glass container

Mix all the oils in container. Apply before going to bed.

Eyelash Conditioner

½ tsp coconut oil
¼ tsp Amla oil
¼ tsp grapeseed oil
¼ tsp of dried Nettle
0.25 oz container

-Mix all the ingredients in container.
-Heat in the microwave for 15 seconds or until it boils. Let the nettle steep in the oil for 30 minutes.
-Strain the mixture, using a fine strainer or a coffee paper filter. Try to strain the oil into a similarly small recipient.
-Once the oil mixture has cooled, proceed to apply it to your lashes. You can use your fingertips or a small plastic lash mascara brush.

Under-eye Dark Circles!

1 tsp Mint leaves
½ a cup of Milk.

Boil milk and let mint leaves steep.
Strain the mixture. Freeze to make ice cubes.
Rub daily on the eyes area.

Puffy Eyes!

Use ice cold tea bags as cold compressions to reduce under-eye bags and puffiness.

Dark Circles!

To lighten dark circles under your eyes, cut slices of potato and apply to eyelids for 15-20 minutes.
Rinse with warm water.

Eye Cream

1 Tbsp lanolin
2 tsp almond oil
2 tsp wheat germ oil
1 tsp apricot oil
2 tsp purified water

Melt the oils and lanolin in a double boiler until the mixture is liquid but not overheated. Warm the water in a separate container to the same temperature as the oil mixture and slowly trickle the water into the oils. Stir constantly until cool and spoon into sterilized jars and cap immediately

Ingredient Talk

Camphor oil

Only the white camphor oil is used and has a clear and fresh smell. The brown and yellow camphor is toxic and carcinogenic since it contains safrole and is not used in aromatherapy. It is powerful oil and should be used with care. It is not really used in aromatherapy as it is classed as a convulsant and neurotoxin. Although very small amounts of camphor oil would be included in any formulation, it does have value in fighting inflammatory conditions and reducing redness, making it useful for treating acne, burns and sore chapped hands.

Grapeseed Oil

Grapeseed oil comes from the common grape vine (Vitis vinifera). It is quickly and deeply absorbed by the skin, making it suitable for light massage of delicate or oily skin. It is odorless and almost colorless and is therefore an ideal base to which essential oils could be added. It is very rich in vitamin C and anti-oxidants.

Coconut Oil

The oil is obtained from the pressing of coconuts. It has softening and moisturizing effects. It is an excellent ingredient in hair care products.

Nettle

(Urtica dioica) rich in minerals, this is one of nature's finest spring tonics. It is useful as a wash for a dry, flaking scalp.

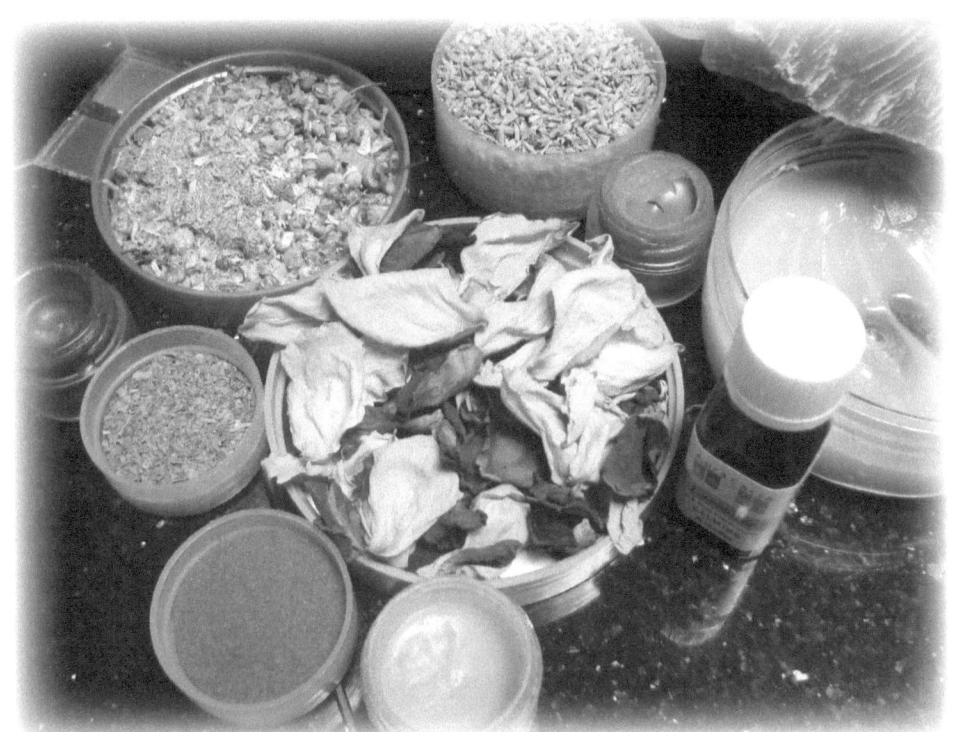

Lips

Lip Balm

.25 oz glass container
½ tsp of Grapeseed Oil or Castor Oil or any other preferred base oil
½ tsp of beeswax
¼ tsp of honey
5 drops of Essential oil of spearmint or peppermint (for flavor)
5 drops of Essential oil of Tea Tree Oil (to treat cold sores)
Optional: ½ tsp of Cocoa butter

-Place all ingredients in 0.25 oz. glass container.
-Microwave for 20 seconds or until you see that all materials have melted
 and it is boiling for the first time.

-Pull out of the microwave taking care not to burn your fingertips.
-Place in the freezer for 30 minutes to 1 hour. Mixture should be hardened.
-Apply.

To Add Color to your Lip Balm

You can use either ¼ tsp of your favorite lipstick color and melt it along with all the other ingredients listed to make Lip Balm, or you can use natural pigments derived from herbs and spices as listed in the next page. With this formula you may also be able to make cream eyeliners or eyebrow cream color. Please revert to the eye section and use the oils for eyes, but think of giving your creams color the same way we are adding color to lipbalm.

Natural Tinting Herbs for lip balms

Alkanet Root Powder—Gives a natural dark red to purple tint. The powdered roots are used to infuse oil with its red, burgundy color. (Use about 2 Tbsp powder per cup of oil) It can be used in soap or other formulations containing oil.
Annato seed—For a deep orange color. It can be infused in oil to tint skin care products naturally. Use 1 tsp of Annato seeds per cup of oil to get dark orange oil. Olive oil or any vegetable oil is a good choice for this. Use as needed in Creams, lotions, soaps, bath salts, bath bombs and lip balms.
Paprika powder—For a rich orange color. Make infused oil and used the strained oil infusion for all formulations containing oil.

Other Natural Tinting Herbs

Henna Leaf Powder—For a rich orange color. The infused oil can be used to create a natural color for your toiletries and soap. It's cooling, astringent, anti-fungal and anti-bacterial for skin and hair.
Sandalwood Red Powder—It is often used in soap making to yield a dark maroon to purple color. For this purpose try using 1 tsp of Red Sandalwood powder per 1 lb. of soap.

Turmeric Powder—For a Yellow color. Used for skin preparations and other formulations. It is an anti-bacterial, good to treat skin infections, boils, wounds and burns.

Fruit Fiber Cranberry—Can be used to add natural color to natural scrubs and soaps.

Fruit Fiber Kiwi—For beige color.

Dried raspberry fruit seed powder-To give a pinky color. Adds color to natural soaps and scrubs.

Nettle Stinging Powder—For Green. To achieve a natural green color in soaps. Make an oil infusion and use the strained oil.

Parsley Powder—Green colorant for soaps. Parsley is soothing, cleansing and detoxifying when added to baths and skin care products. Helps open up and cleanse the pores. Add Parsley powder to bath teas, milk baths, bath salts and detox body wraps.

Home-made Lip Gloss

Mix 1 tsp liquid Glycerine
½ tsp Almond Oil.

Glide over your lips for a natural shine!
Never throw away roll-on perfume containers, or lip glosses, rather wash them and pour in your new Home made lip gloss.

Soft Lips

2 tsp coconut oil,
2 tsp lemon juice
3 drops of lemon oil
1 tsp bees wax

Mix all ingredients. Heat in glass container in microwave for 1 min. or until it melts.
pour into a glass jar of desired store.

Rosemary Lip Repair

1 Tbsp beeswax
2 Tbsp sesame oil
1 Tbsp wheat germ oil
1 tsp almond oil
10 drops rosemary essential oil
2 vitamin E capsules
1/2 tsp glycerin

Melt the wax in the oils listed above. Add the vitamin E, the rosemary essential oil and glycerin. Blend all. Pot the mixture quickly while soft.

Ingredient Talk

Honey

The sweet syrup made by bees is an excellent humectant for moisturizing the skin, and also has antiseptic properties.

Peppermint Essential oil

Peppermint is known for its decongestant, stimulating and refreshing properties. Menthol, which is usually obtained from peppermint, has decongestant and cooling properties.

Tea Tree Essential Oil

Tea Tree essential oil is extracted from the leaves of the tree (Melaleuca alternifolia) which is native to Australia. Its excellent germicidal and antifungal properties give it a wide range of uses, including the treatment of colds, flu, herpes, thrush, athlete's foot, warts, and other skin infections.

Cocoa Butter

(Theobroma Cacao/ Cacao chocolate nut tree) Cocoa Butter is the fat that is obtained from the roasted seeds of the cocoa bean, the fruit of this tree. The butter contains stearic, palmitic and oleic acids, and it is used as an emollient and conditioning agent.

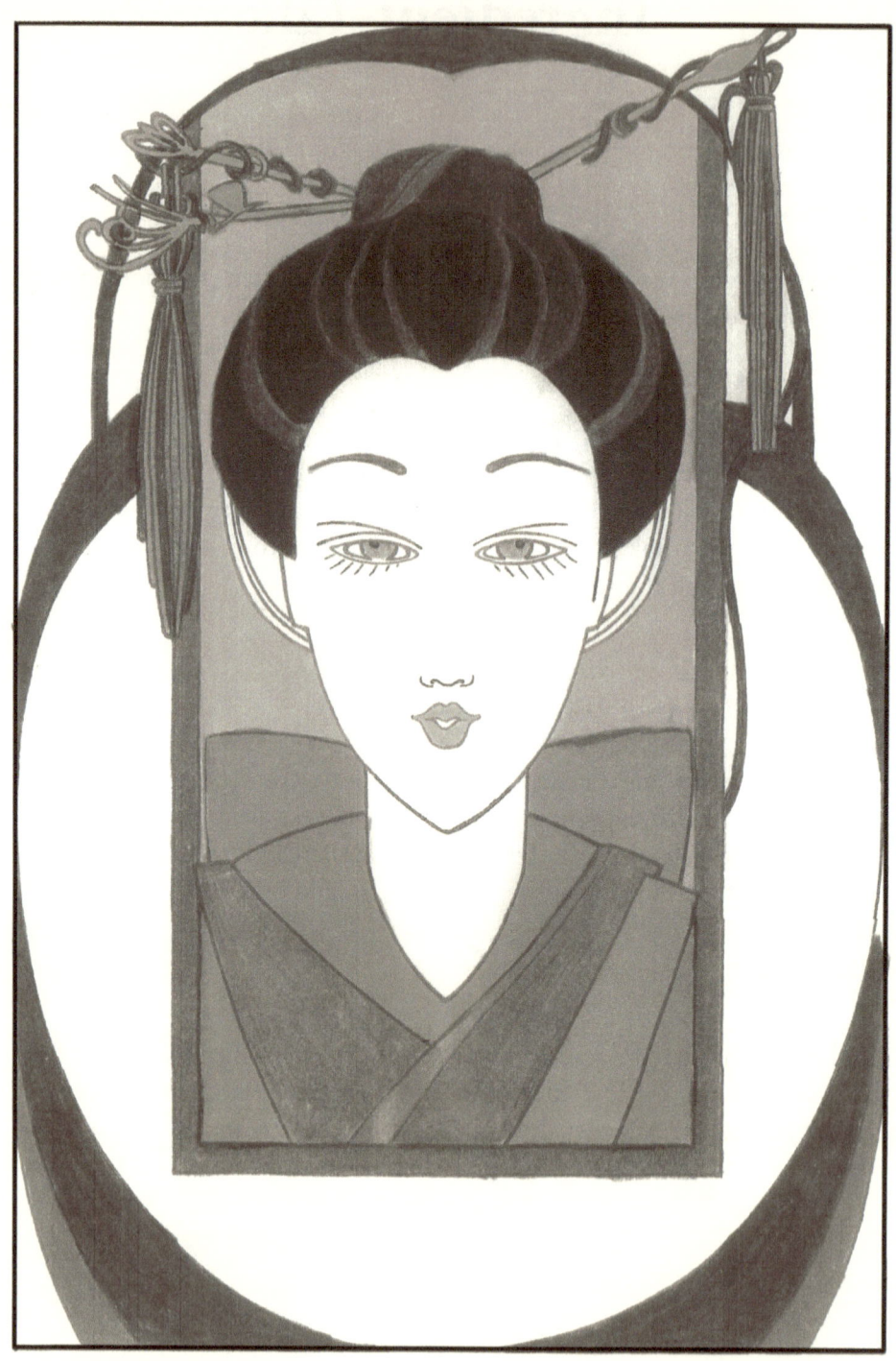

FACE

Black tea or Camellia Sinensis Cream

0.25 glass container
1 tea bag of Lipton Black tea
2 Tbsp Grapeseed oil
1 Tbsp Beeswax

-In the glass container, pour the grapeseed oil and heat up the herbs contained in the tea bag. This can be done directly in the microwave for 20 seconds or until first boil.
-Take the mixture out of the microwave making sure not to burn yourself. Let it cool a bit, and strain using a metal strainer, cheese cloth, or a coffee filter.
-Take the strained oil and put in the beeswax. Heat the mixture in the microwave until the beeswax is fully melted. Take out carefully.
-Cover.
-Place in the freezer for 30 minutes to an hour to harden.

This cream promotes Blood flow from the caffeine it contains. It also repairs sun damaged skin for it contains Fluoride. It is a very good skin repair cream, because it is anti-oxidant rich.

Lavander and Lemon Moisturizers

This moisturizer has antiseptic and healing properties suitable for oily or problem skin.

1 Tbsp of Lavender dried flowers
3 Tbsp of Grape seed oil
1 tsp of beeswax
¼ tsp of cocoa butter
10 drops of lemon essential oil
1 baby food empty glass jar

-In a glass jar, pour the grapeseed oil and the lavender flowers.

-Heat the mixture in the microwave until the oil boils.

-Take out and let the herbs steep in the oil for a while, when you notice that the oil has a strong Lavender aroma, strain the mixture.

-Put the lavender oil into the baby food jar add the pellets of beeswax and cocoa butter.

-Place in the microwave until the beeswax and cocoa butter melt.

-Take mixture out being careful not to burn yourself.

-Add the lemon essential oil drops. Cap the jar. Shake sideways and place in the freezer.

-Leave it there for 30 min. or until it has hardened.

Rose Facial Oil

Exquisite oil suitable for delicate skin. It could be applied at night for a luxurious and rejuvenating facial massage or it could be applied as conditioning oil after the shower, when skin is damp.

1 oz. glass or plastic recipient with lid
6 tsp grapeseed oil
5 drops of rose absolute essential oil
5 drops of patchouli essential oil
5 drops of geranium essential oil

Mix all the ingredients together. Cap. Shake before use.

Wheat germ Ointment

This is a moisturizing and soothing balm for dry skin, wrinkles, stretch marks and surface sores. Useful in minor burns. May relief minor muscular aches and pains, cramping, soreness and muscular backache.

4 oz.. wheat germ oil
½ tsp of vitamin E
½ Tbsp of Beeswax
1 tsp of Cocoa Butter
½ Tbsp of Aloe Vera oil
5 drops of geranium rose essential oil
5 drops of lavender essential oil.
4.4 oz. glass or plastic recipient

-In a glass container pour the wheat germ oil, vitamin E, cocoa butter, beeswax and aloe Vera oil.
-Heat in the microwave until the beeswax and cocoa butter have melted.
-Take out with caution of heat! If you desired to use a plastic container, pour onto the plastic container and add the drops of essential oil. Cap.
-Shake sideways. Use a Kitchen mitten to handle for the container is going to be extremely hot!
-Place in the freezer and leave there for 30 minutes or until it solidifies into an ointment.

Chamomile Cream for sensitive skin

2 Tbsp grapeseed oil
2 Tbsp jojoba oil
1 Tbsp grated beeswax
1 400 IU Vitamin E capsule (optional)
60 mlts rosewater
5 drops chamomile essential oil
5 drops rose essential oil
3 drops grapefruit-seed extract (optional)

In a double boiler warm the oils and add the beeswax. Gently heat the oils and wax until the wax has melt. Do not overheat. Add the vitamin E

capsule content (acts as a preservative), and then stir in the rosewater slowly-trickle it in. Keep stirring the cream until you are sure it has all emulsified and then add the essential oils and grapefruit seed extract (which acts as a preservative and will give the product a shelf life of up to two years)

Citrus & Lavender Moisturizer

2 Tbsp grapeseed oil
2 Tbsp jojoba oil
1 Tbsp grated beeswax
1 400IU capsule Vitamin-E (optional)
60mls aloe vera gel
3 drops grapefruit seed extract (optional)
5 drops lavender essential oil
5 drops grapefruit essential oil

Follow the instructions as for the sensitive skin 'Chamomile Cream' recipe.

Revitalizing Cream for mature skin

3 Tbsp almond oil
1 Tbsp coconut oil
1 Tbsp grated beeswax
1 400IU capsule Vitamin-E (optional)
60mls rosewater
3 drops neroli ess. oil
3 drops sandalwood essential oil
3 drops grapefruit seed extract (optional)

Follow the instructions as per sensitive skin 'Chamomile Cream' recipe.

Apricot Rose Cream Dry/Combination/Normal Skin

2 Tbsp almond oil
2 Tbsp apricot kernel oil
4 gms beeswax
30 mlts. Rosewater
1/2 tsp borax (helps to emulsify & preserve)
2 vitamin E capsules
10 drops essential oil of choice

Mix the almond and apricot Kernel oils and put in the beeswax shavings, heat this mixture until wax is melted. Dissolve the borax into the rosewater and slowly add to the wax/oil mixture. Add the contents of the vitamin E capsules when the mixture is below 50 degrees Celsius. Spoon into sterilized jars and cap immediately.

Citrus Smooth Skin

Take a cup of sugar, add concentrate of orange or lemon juice.
Lather your body and face. Scrub the whole body and face with this mixture.
Rinse generously with warm water. You'll get a delightful smooth skin.

Mango Satin Smooth Skin!

When you eat a Mango, don't throw the peels. Dry the peels. Powder the peels. Add 1 tsp milk powder and rub all over.
Wash off after 5 minutes for a satin finish!

Vitamin A Cream

1 TBS lanolin
15 g beeswax
2 TBS olive oil
1 TBS cod liver oil
2 teaspoons unperfumed talc

Mix the lanolin with the beeswax and heat until the beeswax is melted. You can choose a double boiler for this. Do not overheat. Heat the olive and cod-liver oil and mix well with the talc. Add to the lanolin/wax mixture and stir well. Pot into sterilized containers and cap immediately.

Cocoa Butter Moisturizer for Face or Body

This is a wonderful moisturizer for dry skin and it can be use daily.

1 Tbsp Cocoa Butter
2/3 cup or 5 oz. of Grapeseed oil
6 drops of essential oil of sandalwood, fennel or geranium.

-In a glass container pour the grapeseed oil and the pellets of cocoa butter.
-Place in the Microwave and heat until cocoa butter has melted.
-Pull out of the microwave very careful not to burn yourself with the hot container.
-Place in desired container if different from the one the mixture melted.
-Add the drops of essential oil. Cap. Shake sideways.
-Put in freezer to harden.
-Apply.

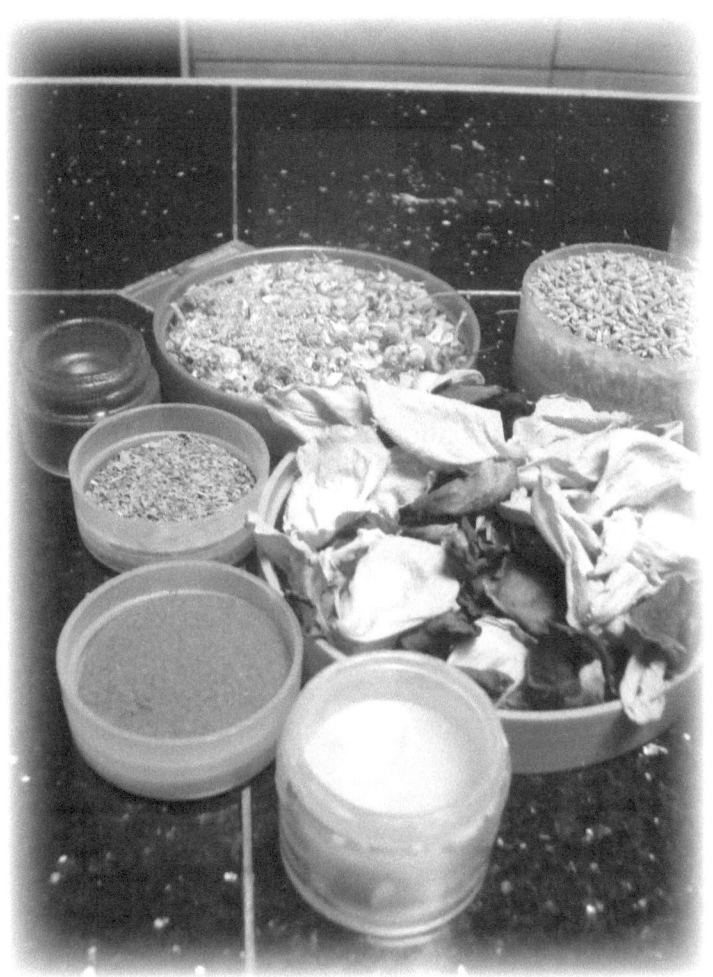

CLEANSING

Fennel Cleansing Cream

2 Tbsp crushed fennel seeds
1/2 cup of buttermilk

Heat the milk and fennel seeds in the boiler for half an hour.
Do not bring to a boil. Turn off the heat and let it cool for two hours.
Use as a cleansing cream. It is good for 2 wks if refrigerated.

Rosewater & Glycerin Cleanser for Sensitive Skin

Here is a very simple recipe for a sensitive skin cleanser that is also suitable for normal and dry skin types.

125ml rosewater
125ml vegetable liquid glycerin
2 drops rose essential oil.

Mix all the ingredients together in a glass bottle and shake well. Apply this liquid cleanser, rubbing it over your face and rinse with warm water.

Aromatherapy Cleansing Cream for Dry Skin

60 mlts rosewater
60 mlts vegetable liquid glycerin
60 mlts Aloe Vera gel
5 drops Palma Rosa oil
2 drops rose oil.

Combine all the ingredients in a glass bottle and shake well.

Herbal Cleansing Lotion for Normal Skin

60mls witch hazel
60mls rosewater
1 tsp dried elder flowers
1 tsp dried calendula flowers
1 tsp dried chamomile
60mls liquid glycerin

Steep the herbs in the witch hazel and rosewater in a jar for a week. Strain and then add the glycerin. Decant into a glass bottle and shake well.

Aromatherapy Cleanser for Normal Skin

60mls rosewater
60mls liquid glycerin
60 ml Aloe Vera juice
10 drops lavender oil

Mix all the ingredients together in a glass bottle and shake well.

Orange Blossom Cleansing Cream for Mature Skin

2 Tbsp jojoba oil
1 Tbsp almond oil
1 Tbsp coconut oil
1 Tbsp grated beeswax
1 400IU Vitamin E capsule (optional)
80mls rosewater
3 drops neroli or petitgrain essential oil
3 drops palma rosa essential oil
3 drops grapefruit seed extract (optional)

Follow the instructions as explained in the sensitive skin 'Chamomile Cream' recipe.

* The following recipe needs to be stored in the fridge. This recipe is enough to last for a week. After that time the product should be disposed of.

Acne & Blemished Skin

Herbal Cleanser

1 tsp dried thyme
1 tsp dried lavender
1 tsp dried calendula flowers
1 tsp dried comfrey
60mls rosewater
2 Tbsp liquid glycerin

Steep the herbs in the witch hazel and rosewater for a week, shaking daily. Strain the mixture and add the glycerin. To use, saturate a cosmetic pad with the lotion and wipe over the face.

Herbal Cleansing Milk

125ml plain yoghurt
125mls water
1 Tbsp dried calendula
1 Tbsp dried thyme
2 Tbsp dried comfrey leaf

Make an infusion with the herbs and the water. Leave to stand over night then strain and mix the liquid into the yoghurt.

Aromatherapy Cleanser for Oily Skin

60mls witch hazel
60mls liquid glycerin
60mls aloe Vera gel
1 Tbsp cider vinegar
5 drops grapefruit essential oil
2 drops lemon essential oil

Mix all the ingredients together in a glass bottle and shake well.

MASKS

*The next recipe will not keep for more than a week without refrigeration.

Aromatherapy Facial Mask

2 tsp natural, whole-fat yoghurt
1/2 tsp cosmetic clay
1/2 tsp jojoba oil
2 drops sandalwood
1 drop rose essential oil

Mix all the ingredients together in a small bowl. Apply to skin after cleansing. Leave on for up to 20 minutes. Rinse and follow with toner and moisturizer.

Normal Skin

*The following recipe must be kept in the fridge. Use within a week.

Aromatherapy facial mask

2 tsp whole-fat natural yoghurt
1/2 tsp cosmetic clay
2 drops lavender essential oil
1 drop geranium essential oil

Mix all the ingredients together and smear over a cleansed face. Leave for 20 minutes, then rinse, tone and moisturize.

Oily Skin

Basic Mask

100g fuller's earth or kaolin clay
2 TBS corn flour
1 TBS finely ground oats
1 TBS finely ground almond meal

Mix all together and store in a tightly covered jar. Mix 1 TBS of the mixture to a soft paste with honey, fruit juice or pulp, vinegar, yoghurt, egg, a herbal infusion or decoction. Spread over your face and leave for 15 minutes.

Peppermint Face Pack

1 tsp of peppermint extract
1 tsp of witch hazel extract
125 grms of brewer's yeast
1 tsp of lemon juice.

Mix all the ingredients together. Apply on the face, forehead and relax by lying horizontally keeping the eyes closed. Leave it for 30 minutes.
Then wash off with lukewarm water containing a little of lemon juice.
This face pack is very good for patchy skin. It is also good for improving blood circulation.

Toners

Orange Flower Toner

1 Tbsp orange flowers
1 tsp rose petals
2 Tbsp Glycerin
1 cup distilled water

-Bring water to a boil and remove from heat.
-Add Herbs and steep for 45 minutes in a covered pot.
-Strain.
-Slowly add glycerin stirring constantly.
-Store.
-Use 1 tsp per application. Shake vigorously before use.

Aloe Vera Toner

This is a good toner for normal to oily skin.

Pure Aloe Vera Gel

NOTE: You can either purchase the Aloe Vera Gel or cut a leaf from the Aloe Vera plant. If you are to cut the leaf from the plant, be careful not to poke yourself with the thorns. Strip all of its skin off and use the gel that is inside the leaf as skin toner.

-Take all the remaining gel of the plant; place it in a glass jar.
-Cover and store in the refrigerator.
-Another use you can give it is to add shine to your hair; you can mix it
  with your shampoo or conditioner.

Rose Toner

This is a good toner for sensitive and dry skin.

1 cup of distilled water
2 Tbsp of rose petals
1 Tbsp of Glycerin

-Bring water to a boil and remove from heat.
-Add Rose petals and steep for 45 minutes in a covered pot. Strain.
-Slowly add glycerin stirring constantly.
-Store.
-Use 1 tsp per application. Shake vigorously before use.

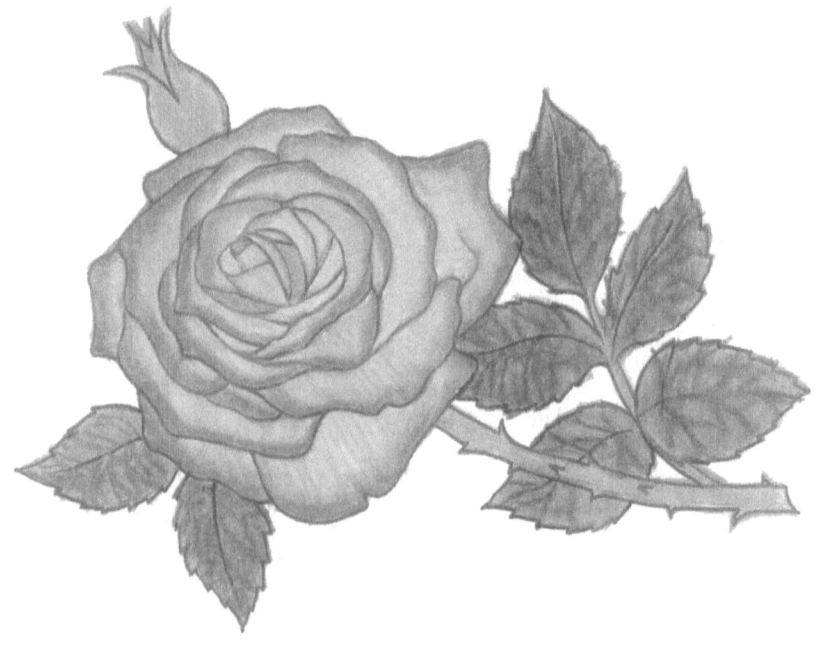

Rosemary Astringent Lotion

2 Tbsp of Rosemary powder
1 Tbsp of Orange peels
2 Tbsp of Lemon peels
1/2 tsp of Sodium Benzoate
1/4 Brandy
30 Mint leaves
1 cup of Rose water.

Soak the lemon and orange peels, mint leaves and rosemary powder in boiling rose water and Brandy for 1 hour. Mix in the Sodium Benzoate. Strain.
Bottle and refrigerate. It's good for a long time!

Aromatherapy Toner

1 tsp witch hazel
5 drops lavender essential oil
5 drops rose essential oil
250 ml rosewater.

Mix all the ingredients together in a glass bottle and shake well. Apply to skin after cleansing with a cosmetic pad.

DRY SKIN

Herbal Toner

125 mlts witch hazel
125 mlts rosewater
1 tsp liquid glycerin
1 tsp dried chamomile
1 tsp dried calendula flowers
1 tsp dried rose petals

Mix all the ingredients in a glass jar and allow to steep for a week. After the week is up, strain the liquid to remove the dried herbs. Decant into a glass bottle and apply to face after cleansing with cotton wool.

Aromatherapy Toner

1 tsp witch hazel
20 drops sandalwood essential oil
1 tsp liquid glycerin
250 mlts rosewater

Mix all the ingredients together in a glass bottle. Apply to skin after cleansing with cotton wool.

Simple Toner for Normal Skin

125mls water
1 tsp witch hazel
10 drops lavender oil

Mix all the ingredients together and shake well.

Aromatherapy Astringent for oily skin

250mls witch hazel
10 drops juniper essential oil
10 drops lavender essential oil

Mix ingredients together in a glass bottle and shake well.

Herbal Astringent for oily skin

250mls witch hazel
2 tsp dried yarrow
1 tsp dried sage
1 tsp dried peppermint
1 tsp dried comfrey

Mix all the ingredients well. Allow to steep for two weeks, shaking daily. Strain and decant into a glass bottle.

Calendula Skin Tonic for all skin types

1 cup fresh calendula flowers
2 cups boiling water
1/4 tsp tincture of benzoin

Mix the flowers and water together in a heatproof bowl. Allow to stand in a warm place for 4 hours. Strain and bottle. Add the tincture and Shake well.

Pep-Up Astringent

1 teacup fresh peppermint
1/2 teacup fresh calendula flowers
Boiling water to cover
1/2 cup witch hazel
1 teaspoon tincture of benzoin
4 drops peppermint oil

Chop the herbs finely, mix together and cover with boiling water. Leave for four hours. Strain and add the witch hazel and benzoin and mix well. Bottle.

Cool in Summer

To keep your cool in summer, avoid sugary foods and drinks. Instead, drink plenty of fresh fruit juices and coconut water.

NOTE: **Tincture of benzoin is the suggested preservative for these cosmetic recipes, but you can use grapefruit seed extract if you wish.**

Exfoliants or Scrubs

Honey and Sugar scrub

For the face use: 1 Tbsp of Honey
                   1 tsp of sugar

-Mix together.
-Apply and massage in soft circular movement all over your face, taking
 care of sensitive skin like the under eyes and the eyelids.
-Rinse with lukewarm water when done.

Herbal Ubtan

This scrub has a gentle softening and cleansing effect.

Mix together equal parts of:

Ground coriander
Ground cumin
Ground fenugreek
Ground liquorice
Chick pea powder

-For **oily combination or blemished skin**, mix the blend to a paste with
 yogurt or diluted lemon juice.
-For **dry or mature skin,** mix the blend to a paste with milk or cream.
-For **normal skin**, mix the blend to a paste with rose water or water.

Once you have the desired paste consistency, rub it into your face using
small circular movements. Massage off with warm water followed by cool
water.

Ingredient Talk

Lavender

(Lavandula Agustifolia) This herb is calming and healing for delicate and sensitive skins. Lavender Essential oil, with its sweet fragarance, is one of the most used oils. It has balancing effect on the nervous system, it can help relieve headache, and prevent insomnia. It is pleasant to use in massage and baths. The oil has antiseptic properties that could be used in the healing of burns, wounds, bites, dermatitis and any inflammation of the skin.

Lemon

(Citrus Limon) The fruit is an astringent and toner; it decreases the production of sebum. It's a great source of Vitamin C and it could be used on the hair to enhance blonde highlights. Lemon Essential oil is expressed from the peel of ripe lemons. It is highly antiseptic and has an astringent effect on the skin. It may be used to treat boils, broken capillaries, greasy skin, herpes and insect bites.

Rose

Pink and red rosebuds may be used for their cooling and soothing action. They may be used as an infusion for itchy, inflamed or sunburned skin. Rose essential oil is an exquisite oil produced from "damask Rose" and " Provence Rose or Cabbage Rose". It is a cooling and soothing oil, used to treat stress related conditions and menstrual problems. It is beneficial for dry, inflamed and mature skins.

Patchouli

(Pogostenum cablin) Patchouli essential oil is distilled from the dried leaves of the Pogostenum Cablin plant. It is used in perfumery for its fixative properties. Patchouli is claimed to be an aphrodisiac, and it may be used in skin care to reduce scarring and to treat oily and problem skin.

Geranium

(Pelargonium graveolens) rose geranium, sweet scented geranium. Geranium essential oil is produced from the leaves of this species. It is a cooling and calming oil, useful in the treatment of anxiety and tension. It has a balancing effect on the skin, making it suitable for dry, oily or problem skin. It is a very pleasant oil to use in massage and bath.

Vitamin E

Tocopherol, a form of vitamin E, usually extracted from soya oil. It is used as an antioxidant in cosmetics and toiletries. It is non-toxic and non-sensitizing. It is also known as vitamin E acetate.

Aloe Vera

A mucilage, known as Aloe Vera juice is extracted from the plant. It is used externally for its soothing, cooling and anti-irritant properties. It is excellent for treating burns, and insect bites.

Sandalwood

(Santalum album) Sandalwood essential oil is distilled from the wood of the tree. It has long been regarded as having aphrodisiac properties. Sandalwood is particularly beneficial for dry skin.

Fennel

(Foeniculum vugare) Fennel essential oil is steam-distilled from the crush seeds of F. vulgare var. dulce, a plant cultivated in the Mediterranean Europe. It has a very sweet fresh smell, reminiscent of aniseed. It is widely used to freshen the breath and to treat conjunctivitis.

Shea Butter

Also known as Shea nut butter is a natural butter obtained from the fruit of the tree Butyrospernum parkii.

Fuller's Earth

An absorptive clay consisting of fine siliceous material, used in facemasks to draw out impurities from the skin. It may be used instead of talk.

Orange Flowers

Beneficial to mature and dry skin types.

Glycerin

A colorless, odorless viscous liquid with a very sweet taste, technically known as glycerol. It is a form of alcohol that is used as a solvent, sweetener and humectant in cosmetics. It helps to prevent creams from drying out.

Coriander

(Coriandurum Sativum) It is a natural deodorant and aphrodisiac.

Comfrey Root

Comfrey (Symphytum officinale) or "knitbone" the old country name, tells about the great healing power of this herb. Used externally as a compress, it helps fractured bones to mend and cuts, ulcers, and bruises to heal with minimal scar formation.

Lemon Grass

(Cymbopogon citratus) lemon grass essential oil is extracted by distillation from this grass. It has a strong, fresh grass and lemony scent. Lemon grass is strong antibacterial oil, useful for treating problem skin, open pores and acne. It is a good insect repellent.

Apricot Kernel oil

This oil is expressed from the kernels of the fruit of his tree.

Calendula

(Calendula officinalis) or Marigold is a spasmolytic, anti-hemorrhagic, emmenagogic, vulnerary, stypic and antiseptic. It is a most useful first aid remedy. Used externally as a wash or cream it is good to heal burns and sores, while the crushed leaves will prevent bleeding and is itself antiseptic. The remedy may also be used externally for varicose veins, ulcers and hemorrhoids, and applied as an eye lotion for the treatment of conjunctivitis. Calendula ointment is used as a soothing and healing treatment for irritated or inflamed skin, for rashes and for eczema.

Problem Skin

Advice for Dry Skin

Dry skin has a matt texture, tends to flake and looks white or grey in patches. It is often aggravated because the sebaceous glands are lazy or the skin has been over-exposed to wind, sun or sea. Central heating also worsens dry skin.

-Avoid all astringents or cosmetics that contain alcohol.
-Even for your cleansing routine or make-up remover use oil or butter. Rub olive, almond or jojba oil or Shea butter into your face to remove make-up and then remove oil in the face with a damp towel or damp cotton.
-Scrub off dead skin gently and not so often. Once a month is enough.
-Do not consume a lot of sugar or drink alcohol.
-Do not smoke cigarettes or passive smoke.

-Do not consume a lot of caffeinated drinks.
-Moisturize your skin more during the winter months.
-Drink 8 cups of water a day.
-Eat your fruits and vegetables.
-Do not eat, too much red meat. Eat only twice a week, leaving 2 days in between of full vegetarianism.
-Do not abuse sun bathing. Protect your skin from sunlight using sun glasses, or hats.
-Exercise often.
-Be ware of the ingredients in cosmetics you have been using in your skin before.

Have you noticed that the products you buy designed for your dry skin never seem to solve the problem? You get some temporary relief after the intital application, but after a while you just have to keep using more and more for the same result? The reason for this is because most of the cosmetics available on the market are made from mineral oil, a cheap oil derived from petrolatum which has the catch-22 ability-it will relieve the skin and restore moisture, but at the same time it depletes the skin of moisture so you have no choice but to use more to get the same result. Making your own creams puts you in control of what you smear over your body.

Treatments

-Apply almond oil to the skin while damp, after the shower.
-Rub cool melon on the face.

<u>Dry Skin Mask</u>

1 egg yolk
1 tsp. honey

Mix together, and spread over the face and neck. Leave on for 20 minutes and then rinse off.

Dry Skin Scrub

1 tsp chickpea flour or 1 tsp of oatmeal powder
½ Tbsp of Honey

Rub over your skin. Scrub of dead skin cells. Rinse thoroughly.

Skin Lightening

1. Apply a mixture of Sandalwood paste and Rose water on your face daily.

2. Make a fine paste of ground Almonds and Rose water and apply it on neck and face. This brings a glow on the face.

3. Soak raw Potatoes for ten minutes in cold water. Rub slices over the face, neck and hands.

4. Soak 4 Almonds every night. Next morning, remove their skin, grind them till they become fine.

Add 1 tsp of Gram Flour, 1 tsp of Milk and 4 drops of Lime Juice. Make a paste and apply on face. Massage the face gently.

5. Make a mixture of grated Cucumber and Coconut water to apply on face.

6. Mixture of Turmeric powder and Sandalwood paste should be applied daily on face for the glow!

Oily Skin Advice

It is a result of overactive sebaceous glands. It shines in patches, is prone to spots and does not hold on to make-up. It comes with enlarged pores and an oily scalp.

-Wash your face often. At least 5 times a day with cold water.
-Wash face with Fuller's Earth soap or a soap made out of glycerin and lemon essential oil, or any other astringent essential oil.
-Use a clay mask in problem spots.

-Do not use make-up cosmetics that are oily . . . . foundations, and creams that may clog more your pores, and may even give you an oilier look.

-Use transluscent powder over clean skin, in my opinion, it will reduce the shine, even the tone, and will let your skin breath better. Do it lightly, and hopefully use powder derived from organic sources.

-Lower your cholesterol consumption, do not eat pork, or deep fried foods, lower consumption of butter.

-Drink 8 cups of water a day at least.

-Do not touch your skin too much.

-Increase your fruit and vegetable intake.

Treatments

-Make a mask made from Almond and Oatmeal powder mix with water. Apply twice a week.

-Once a week apply a well beaten egg white and a few drops of lemon juice to your face and neck to tighten the skin and close the pores.

These treatments will not keep. Make the amount necessary for the occasion.

Acne Prone Skin Advice

This condition has a lot to do with overactive sebaceous glands, hormonal activity during puberty, stress or over-worked conditions, and a poor or a bad diet will aggravate the problem.

-Purify your Blood.

1. According to Ayurveda, one bulb of garlic a day, cleanses, renews the blood and regulates the digestion. Cook with garlic, or soak a tooth of garlic in vinegar and eat daily.

2. Drink water. To flush out toxins through urine and help skin keep healthy. It must be water only since drinks containing caffeine, such as tea, coffee and cola have the effect of dehydrating the body.

Blackhead Advice

Blackheads are a mixture of old skin debris cells and bits of keratin, all colored by melanin, the pigment that colors our skin and hair. Good cleansing should stop some blackheads from forming, but the best way to get rid of them is by steaming. Steaming brings them to the surface of the skin from where they can be eased out. Always close the pores with mild astringents such as Witch Hazel afterwards.

A good way to keep skin heads at bay is to rub a wedge of juicy red tomato on face and neck, and leave for about 5 minutes. Tomato is very rich in vitamins A, B, C and E and contains amino acids and salts, such as citrates and tartrates, that give it a sour taste and make it a good astringent for the skin.

Blemishes

These are usually temporary skin irritations caused by long exposure to the sun, wind or an excess of alcohol.

Treatments

A light dab of a mixture of turmeric or sandalwood powder with water, should clear the problem. Both, turmeric and sandalwood have anti-septic properties.

Another remedy to this problem is to use the juice of a grated carrot in your skin. Wipe over the blemished area and rinse off after 30 minutes. Carrots contain high quantities of Vitamin A, and are good for eyes and skin.

<u>Enlarged Pores</u>

These are caused by the over-stretching of pores that then fill with excess oil. It can temporarily be resolved by using astringents, to tone the skin.

Treatments

-Use Buttermilk or watered down yogurt as a daily face wash and rinse with cold water.
-Put Ice-cold cucumber juice on your face and neck, to refresh and tone the skin.

Body

Body Butter

4 oz. grapeseed oil or any other base oil of your preference.
2-3 tea bags of chamomile tea or dried 2 Tbsp of dried chamomile flowers
2 Tbsp of dried lavender flowers
1 double boiler pot
1 glass measuring cup
1 Tbsp of Beeswax
1 tsp of Cocoa Butter (optional)
1 4.4-6.6 glass or plastic container with cap
20 drops of essential oil of your choice: ex: 5 drops of tea tree ess. Oil
                                        5 drops of lavender ess. Oil
                                        5 drops of rose ess. Oil
                                        5 drops of whatever else . . . .

-Place water in bottom of double boiler and pour the oil along with herbs in the
 top pot.
-Cover with a lid. Let the water boil. The oil in the top pot will draw the aroma
 and properties from the herbs.
-Once the oil smells pleasant, it is ready to be strained.
-Use a metal strainer, cheesecloth or coffee filter to strain the herbs from the oil.
-Pour the oil into the glass measuring cup and add the Beeswax and Cocoa Butte.
-Place in the microwave to heat for 30 seconds or until the beeswax and
 cocoa butter have fully melted.
-Pour the mixture into a recycled glass or plastic container.
-Store
-Add the drops of essential oils. Cap. Shake
 sideways.
-Place into the freezer for 30 minutes or until
 the mixture hardens into
a buttery cream.
-Massage into your skin and Enjoy!!!

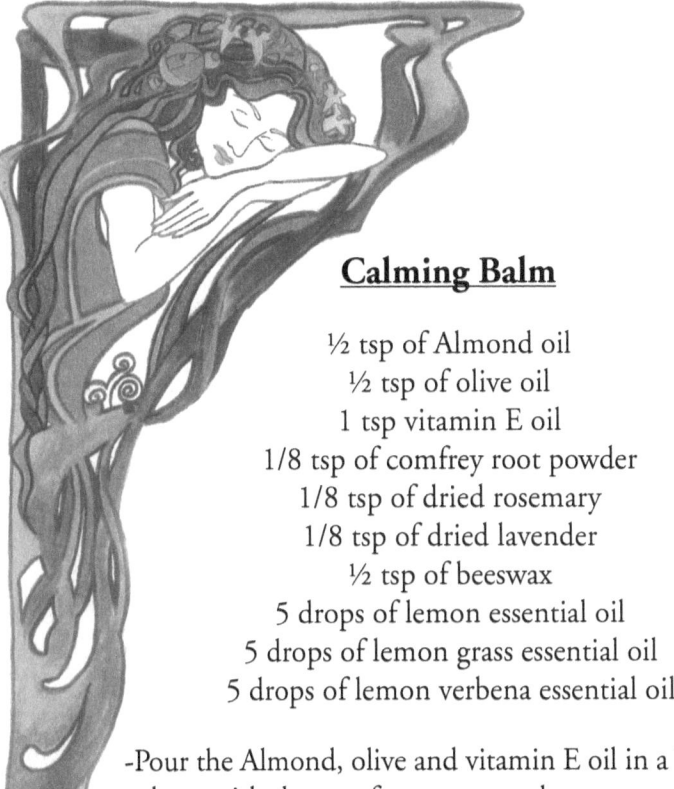

Calming Balm

½ tsp of Almond oil
½ tsp of olive oil
1 tsp vitamin E oil
1/8 tsp of comfrey root powder
1/8 tsp of dried rosemary
1/8 tsp of dried lavender
½ tsp of beeswax
5 drops of lemon essential oil
5 drops of lemon grass essential oil
5 drops of lemon verbena essential oil

-Pour the Almond, olive and vitamin E oil in a baby food glass jar along with the comfrey root powder, rosemary and lavender.
-Place in the microwave for 30 seconds or until oil has been brought to a boil.
Carefully pull out of the microwave and let the herbs steep for 10 minutes.
-Strain the mixture.
-Pour the mixture in same baby food glass jar and add the beeswax.
-Heat in microwave for 20 seconds or until the beeswax has melted.
Bring out of the microwave carefully not to burn yourself. At this point, you can store mixture in a smaller plastic, tin can, or glass container if desired.
-Add the essential oil drops and Cap.
-Place in the freezer for 30 minutes or until mixture hardens. Massage in your body . . .

Nourishing Oil

1 Tbsp of Sweet almond oil
1 Tbsp of Olive oil
1 Tbsp of Avocado oil
1 Tbsp of Jojoba oil
1 Tbsp of Apricot Kernet oil
1 Tbsp of Grapeseed oil
1 Tbsp of Vitamin E oil
8 drops of Geranium Rose essential oil
8 drops of Lavender essential oil

Mix all this oils together. Bottle. Massage into your skin.

Uplifting Oil

1 oz. Grapeseed oil
1 Chamomile tea bag or ½ tsp of dried Chamomile flowers
½ tsp dried rosemary
½ tsp peppermint or 1 peppermint tea bag

-In a double boiler place the water to be boiled in bottom pot and pour the
  oil into the top pot along with the dried herbs.
-Let the water boil and the oil in the top pot get hot. When you feel that
  the oil is charged with the fragrance of the herbs, pull out the pot.
-Strain the mixture.
-Bottle the oil and use as often as you please.

Rose Hand Cream

1 tsp Beeswax
¼ tsp honey
4 Tbsp Almond Oil
4 Tbsp Rose Water
1 glass measuring cup
1 4.4 oz plastic or glass contained with cap

-In the glass measuring cup place the Almond oil, honey and beeswax.
-Microwave for 30 seconds or until the beeswax pellets have melted.
-Take out with care not to burn yourself.
-Add the Rosewater and stir slowly.
-Pour all the mixture into the 4.4 oz. plastic or glass container.
-Cap.
-Shake sideways
-Place into the freezer to cool and harden for 30 to 45 minutes.
-Apply.

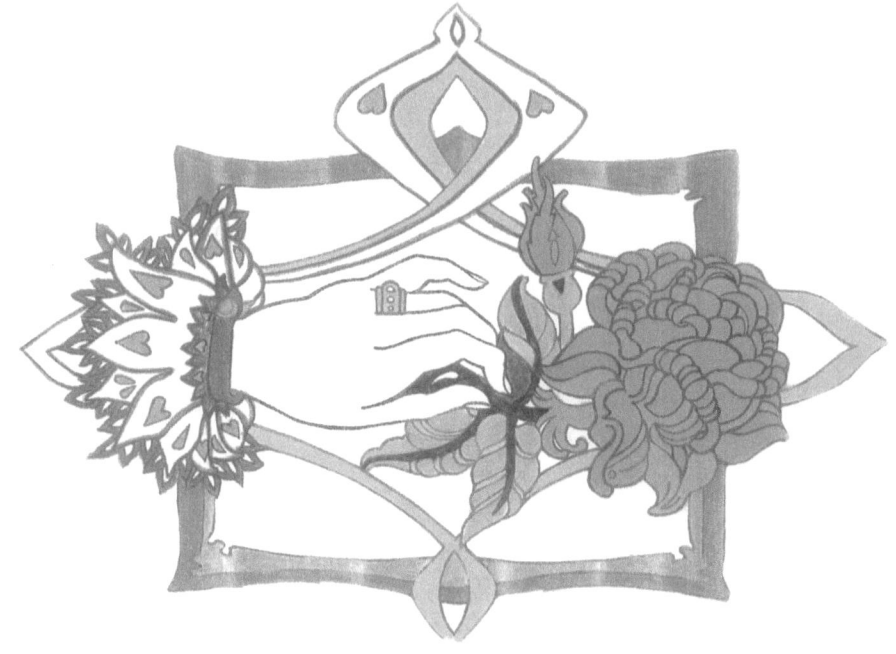

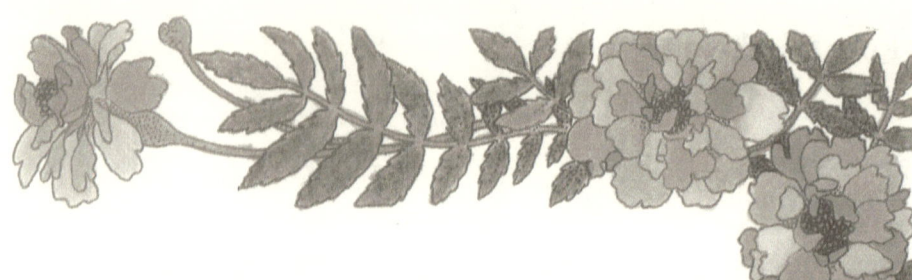

<u>Calendula Ointment</u>

The Calendula flowers or Pot Mary Gold should be harvested at the peak of their bloom and used fresh or carefully dried.

4 oz. grapeseed oil or any other base oil of your preference.
2 Tbsp of dried calendula flowers
1 double boiler pot
1 glass measuring cup
1 Tbsp of Beeswax
4 Tbsp of Cocoa Butter
1 4.4-6.6 glass or plastic container with cap

-Place water in bottom of double boiler and pour the oil along with herbs in the top pot.
-Cover with a lid. Let the water boil. The oil in the top pot will draw the aroma and properties from the herbs.
-Once the oil smells pleasant, it is ready to be strained.
-Use a metal strainer, cheesecloth or coffee filters to strain.
-Pour the oil into the glass measuring cup and add the Beeswax and Cocoa Butter.
-Place in the microwave to heat for 30 seconds or until the beeswax and cocoa butter have fully melted.
-Pour the mixture into your recycled glass or plastic container to store.
-Cap.
-Shake sideways, and place into the freezer for 30 minutes or until the mixture hardens into a buttery cream.
-Massage into your skin and Enjoy!!!

Lotions

Herbal Aftershave Lotion

2 Tbsp calendula flowers, finely chopped
2 Tbsp finely chopped rosemary
2 cups of boiling water
50 ml witch hazel
2 tsp tincture of benzoin

Mix the herbs and boiling water in a jar and leave to steep for 24 hours in a warm place. Strain, add the witch hazel and benzoin, and mix well.

NOTE: **Tincture of benzoin is the suggested preservative for these cosmetic recipe, but you can use grapefruit seed extract if you wish.**

Deodorant Lotion

90ml witch hazel
1 tsp liquid glycerin
30 drops clary sage oil
10 drops lavender essential oil
10 drops thyme essential oil
10 drops patchouli essential oil
5 drops sandalwood essential oil

Blend all the ingredients together in a 125ml bottle. Shake well to mix and leave for four days before using. Shake before use.

Lemon & lavender Hand Softener

30 gms beeswax
100ml almond oil
125mls canola oil
2 TBS glycerin
2 mls lemon essential oil
1 ml lavender essential oil
1 tsp tincture of benzoin.

Mix the almond and canola oils and melt the beeswax within this mixture. Once is melted add the glycerine, tincture of benzoin, and essential oils. Leave to cool at room temperature or in the freezer. Wait for about 30 minutes to harden into a cream.

NOTE: **Tincture of benzoin is the suggested preservative for these cosmetic recipes, but you can use grapefruit seed extract if you wish.**

BABY CARE

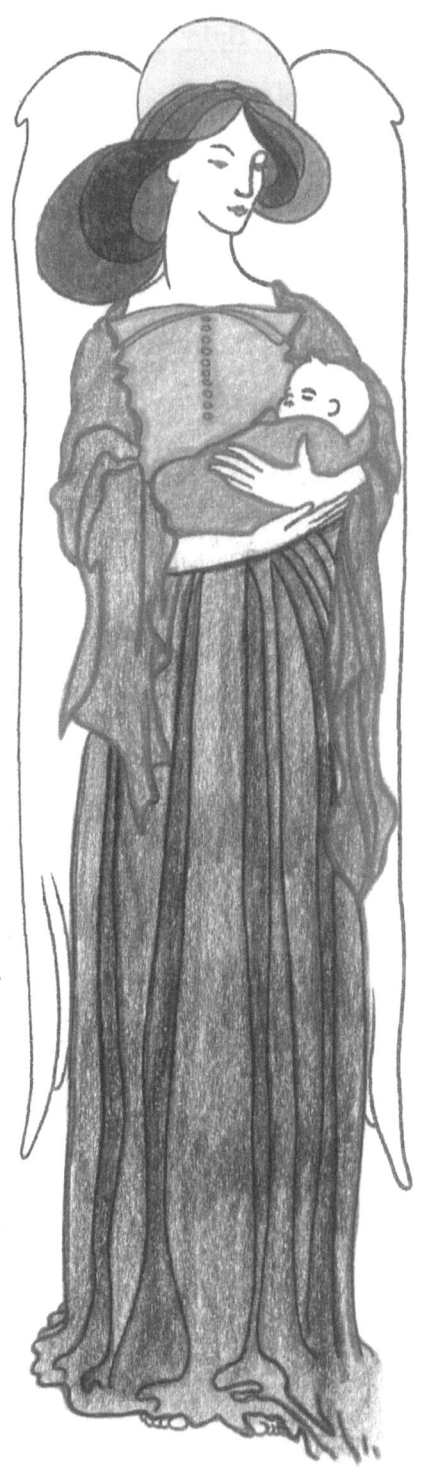

Baby Soap

2 pellets of Solid vegetable glycerin
5-8 drops of lavender essential oil

-Melt the glycerin in a glass measuring
 cup,
you can use your microwave setting the
mixture
to melt for 1 minute or less.
-Take out.
-Pour the lavender drops to the mixture
 and pour mixture
into greased plastic mold.
-Place in the freezer. Take out when solid.

Baby's Bath

I mixed Chamomile tea into his bath . . . .
This relaxes him a lot, and it has a very
pleasant fragrance.

Baby's ointment

4 oz. of grapeseed oil or any other base oil
of your preference.
2-3 tea bags of chamomile tea or dried 2
Tbsp of dried chamomile flowers
2 Tbsp of dried lavender flowers
1 double boiler pot
1 glass measuring cup
1 Tbsp of Beeswax

-In the double boiler place the water to be brought to boil in the bottom
  pot and pour the oil along with herbs in the top pot.
-Cover with a lid. Let the water boil and the oil in the top pot get hot and
  draw the aroma and properties from the herbs.
-Open the top pot and smell to see if the oil has yet saturated with the
  dried herbs aroma. Once the oil smells pleasant, it is ready to be strained.
-Use a metal strainer, cheesecloth or coffee filter to strain the herbs from
  the oil.
-Pour the oil into the glass measuring cup and add the Beeswax and
  Cocoa Butter.
-Place in the microwave to heat for 30 seconds or until the beeswax and
  cocoa butter have fully melted.
-Pour the mixture into your recycled glass or plastic container to store
-Place in the freezer to harden mixture.

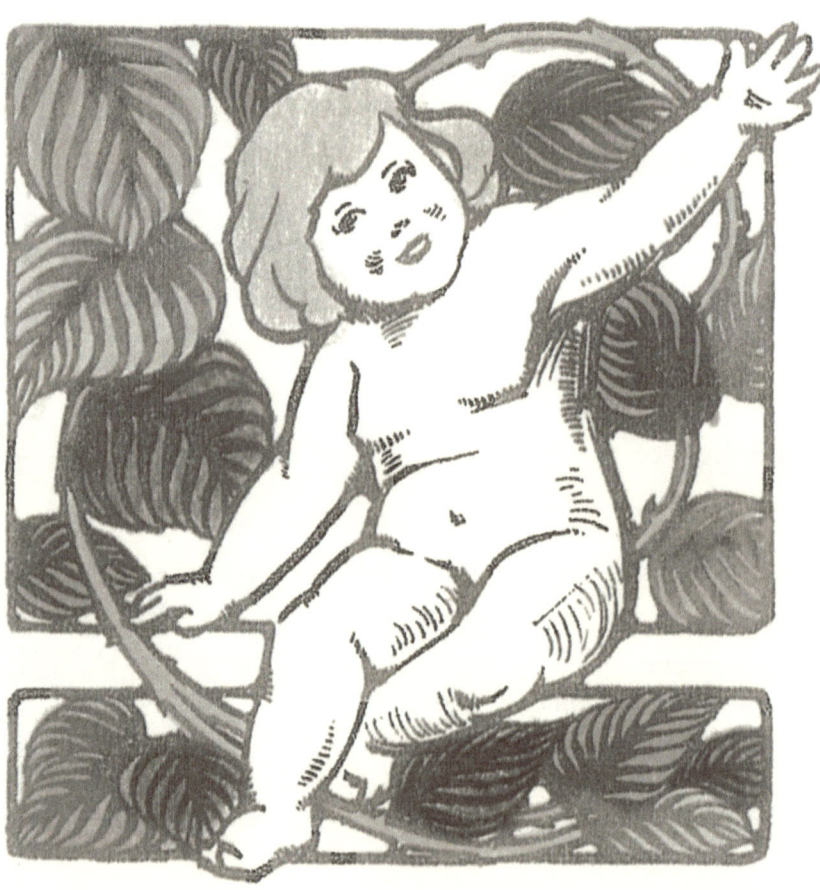

Baby oil

4 oz. of grapeseed oil or any other base oil of your preference.
2-3 tea bags of chamomile tea or dried 2 Tbsp of dried chamomile flowers
2 Tbsp of dried lavender flowers

-In the double boiler place the water to be brought to boil in the bottom
  pot and pour the oil along with herbs in the top pot.
-Cover with a lid. Let the water boil and the oil in the top pot get hot and
  draw the aroma and properties from the herbs.
-Open the top pot and smell to see if the oil has yet saturated with the dried
  herbs aroma. Once the oil smells pleasant, it is ready to be strained.
-Use a metal strainer, cheesecloth or coffee filter to strain the herbs from
  the oil.

NOTE: Never use mineral oil on baby or yourself, it clogs the pores.

Toddler's tangly hair leave-in conditioner and detangler

-Fill up an 8 oz. spritzer bottle with water and add a tsp of oil infused with
  chamomile.
-Close cap, shake, and spritz your son's or daughter curly, tangly hair before
  combing or brushing.
-Comb gently.

BIBLIOGRAPHY

Llewellyn. Llewellyn's 2002 Herbal Almanac. St. Paul, MN:Llewellyn Worldwide. 2002

Mason Haldane. Neal's Yard Remedies: Make your own Cosmetics. London, UK:Aurum Press Ltd. 1997

Tourles, Stephanie. The Herbal Body Book: A Natural Approach to Healthier Hair, Skin and Nails. Pownal, VT: Storey Books.1994

Wright, Janet. Ayurvedic Beauty. London, UK: Aness Publishing Ltd.2002

Clevely Andi, Richmond Katherine, Morris Sallie and Mackley Leslie. Cooking with Herbs and Spices. London, UK: Aness Publishing Ltd. 1997, 2002.

Bharadwaj, Monisha. Beauty Secrets of India: from ayurvedic techniques to exotic adornments.Berkeley, CA: Ulysses Press.

Search Press. The Ultimate Design Book for Crafters. Great Britain: Search Press Ltd. 2006

Mother Earth Aromatherapy. (2004). Natural Skincare-Training Workshop. [Brochure] Perth, Western Australia. Mother Earth Aromatherapy.

Sturt, Cilla. (2002). How Natural is 'Natural'? Wellbeing Body Beautiful; 119-122.

Benhaim, Paul. (2005). Label Gazing. Well Being: 81-85.

Paula Benjoun-The Cosmetics Cop—www.cosmeticscop.com

APPENDIX : WHERE CAN YOU GET THE INGREDIENTS?

Great American Naturals
4121 16th Street N.
St. Petersburg, FL 33703

Extensive line of Herbal care products, essential oils, carrier oils, herbs and spices.

Nature's Finest
6600 Central Avenue
St. Petersburg, FL

oils , herbs, organic produce, health products, essential oils, cocoa butter, ctr.

Michael's Craft Store
2026 66th ST. N
St. Petersburg, FL

Glycerine and Besswax.

Mahal Bazaar
2480 E. Bay Drive Suite C-15
Largo, FL 33771

Herbs and Spices, Dabur Amla oil, Dabur Jasmine Oil.

Deep Foods Inc.
Union, NJ 07083
www.deepfoods.com
Spices and Herbs.

ESSENTIAL OIL	COMBINE WITH	PROPERTIES	EFFECTS
BASIL	Bergamot, chamomile, clary sage, geranium, lavender, lemongrass, marjoram, rose	Nerve Tonic, balancing, reviving strenghtening	Relaxing, Uplifting
BENZOIN	Coriander, cypress, frankincense, jasmine, juniper, lemon, myrrh, rose, sandalwood, spiceoils	Skin irritation, poor circulation	Anti-inflammatory, carminative, astringent
BERGAMOT	Lavender, Melissa, Rosemary	Nerve Tonic	Uplifting
CARDAMON	Bergamot, cedarwood, clove, frankincense, orange, sandalwood, ylang ylang	Digestive tonic, anti-spasmodic, carminative	Tonifying, Calming
CLARY SAGE	Cardamon, coriander, geranium, jasmine lavender, lemon, rose, sandalwood	Nervous system strengthener, aids stress and anxiety	Soothing, sedating
CEDARWOOD	Bergamot, cypress, frankincense, jasmine, juniper, myrrh, neroli, rosemary, sandalwood, vetiver	Warming, regenerating, tonifying, soothing	Balancing
CINNAMON	Clove, eucalyptus, frankincense, lemon, mandarin, orange	Warming, stimulating,	Restorative
CORIANDER	Bergamot, clary sage, frankincense, jasmine, sandalwood	Digestive, mildly warming, tonifying	Aphrodisiac

ESSENTIAL OIL	COMBINE WITH	PROPERTIES	EFFECTS
CLOVE	Bergamot, eucalyptus, lavender thyme	Warming, stimulating, antiseptic	Stimulating, Pain relieving
EUCALYPTUS	Cedarwood, cypress, lavender, lemon, marjoram, pine, tea tree, thyme	Antiseptic, decongestant	Warming, Refreshing
GERANIUM	Bergamot, lavender, lemon, marjoram, neroli, orange, palmarosa, rose, sandalwood	Calming, cooling	Calming, uplifting
GRAPEFRUIT	Citrus oils, clove, cypress, ginger, lavender, neroli, palmarosa, rosemary	Detoxifying, Astringent	Refreshing, Uplifting
JASMINE	Bergamot, clary sage, orange, rose, sandalwood, ylang ylang	Increases self-confidence, anti-depressant	Uplifting, relaxing, aphrodisiac
JUNIPER	Citrus oils, cedarwood, cypress, ginger, lavender, pine, rosemary	Stimulates elimination of toxic fluids	Cleansing
LAVENDER	Geranium, Rosemary	Stress, jetlag, insomnia	Relaxing, Balancing
LEMON	Any	Antiseptic, Astringent	Stimulating

ESSENTIAL OIL	COMBINE WITH	PROPERTIES	EFFECTS
MANDARIN	Citrus oils, spicy oils, clary sage, geranium, lavender, neroli	Digestive, peristalsis	Refreshing, Uplifting
NEROLI	Citrus oils, clary sage, jasmine, lavender, rosemary	Anxiety, Depression, Insomnia	Relaxing, Calming, uplifting
MARJORAM	Bergamot, cypress, eucalyptus, geranium, lavender, orange, rosemary	Relieves aching muscles, period pain	Warming, Relaxing
OLIBANUM	Citrus oils, spice oils, basil, cedarwood, myrrh, neroli, pine, sandalwood, vetiver	Tonifying, Astringent, anti-inflammatory	Aids Meditation
ORANGE	Citrus oils, spice oils, clary sage, geranium, lavender, myrrh, neroli, rosemary	Sluggish digestion, liver detoxifier	Relaxing, Uplifting
PALMAROSA	Bergamot, cedarwood, geranium, mandarin, rose, sandalwood, ylang ylang	Healing, Regenerative	Calming, Uplifting, digestive tonic
PEPPERMINT	Fennel, Orange	Digestive, Antiseptic	Warming, Stimulating
PETIGRATIN	Citrus oils, Clary sage, jasmine, lavender ,rosemary	Nerve Tonic	Uplifting, anti-depressant

ESSENTIAL OIL	COMBINE WITH	PROPERTIES	EFFECTS
ROMAN CHAMOMILE	Clary sage, lavender, lemon, rose	Anti-inflammatory	Sedative
ROSE	Bergamot, chamomile, clary sage, geranium, jasmine, lavender, patchouli	Cooling, relaxing, tonifying	Anti-depressant, aphrodisiac
SANDALWOOD	Bergamot, cedarwood, jasmine, palmarosa, vetiver, ylang ylang	Calming, soothing	Relaxing ,Aphrodisiac, cooling
TEA TREE	Clove, eucalyptus, lavender, lemon, pine, rosemary, thyme	Anti-viral, anti-fungal, antiseptic	Stimulating, tonifying
THYME	Clove, eucalyptus, lavader, lemon, pine	Strongly anti-microbial, strengthens the immune system	Warming, stimulating
VANILLA	Benzoin, sandalwood, spice oils, vetiver	Balsamic	Soothing
VETIVER	Clary Sage, Jasmine, Lavender, Patchouli, Rose, Sandalwood, Ylang ylang	Anti-depressant, aphrodisiac	Sedating, strenghtening
YLANG YLANG	Bergamot, cedarwood, clary sage, jasmine, lemon, rose, sandalwood, vetiver	Treats anxiety, depression, stress, tension	Sedating, calming

CANCER AND ARMPITS

Why breast cancer is usually found near the armpit?

Some time ago, I attended a Breast Cancer Awareness seminar and I asked why the most common area for Breast Cancer was near the armpit.

My question could not be answered at that time.

This e-mail was just sent to me, and I find it interesting that my question has been answered. I challenge you all to rethink your every day use of a product that,could ultimately lead to a terminal illness. As of today, I will change my use.

I showed it to another friend going through chemotherapy & she said she learned this fact in a support group recently.

The leading cause of breast cancer is the use of anti-perspirant . . .

What ???
Yes, *ANTI-PERSPIRANT*.

Most of the products out there are an anti-perspirant/deodorant combination, Deodorant is fine, anti-perspirant is not!

Here's why :—The human body has a few areas that it uses to purge toxins ; behind the knees, behind the ears, groin area, and armpits. The toxins are purged in the form of perspiration.

Anti-perspirant, as the name clearly indicates, prevents you from perspiring, thereby inhibiting the body from purging toxins from below the armpits.

These toxins do not just magically disappear. Instead, the body deposits them in the lymph nodes below the arms since it cannot sweat them out.

Nearly all breast cancer tumors occur in the upper outside quadrant of the breast area. This is precisely where the lymph nodes are located.

Additionally, men are less likely (but not completely exempt) to develop breast cancer prompted by anti-perspirant usage because most of the anti-perspirant product is caught in their hair and is not directly applied to the skin.

Women who apply anti-perspirant right after shaving increase the risk further because shaving causes almost imperceptible nicks in the skin which give the chemicals entrance into the body from the armpit area.

Breast cancer is becoming frighteningly common..

This awareness may save lives.. J.P. Averette